Yoga 101: A Beginner's Step-By-Step Easy to Follow Guide to Understanding and Practicing Yoga

Disclaimer and Terms of Use: Effort has been made to ensure that the information in this book is accurate and complete, however, the author and the publisher do not warrant the accuracy of the information, text and graphics contained within the book due to the rapidly changing nature of science, research, known and unknown facts and internet. The Author and the publisher do not hold any responsibility for errors, omissions or contrary interpretation of the subject matter herein. This book is presented solely for motivational and informational purposes only.

Table of Contents

Introduction

Exercise is one of the primary ways to maintain our health and wellbeing. With the advancement of medicine and modern science man discovered the reasons behind his diseases and illnesses that overcome his life. At present people realize the fact that poor lifestyle and poor food habits are one of the major reasons behind the countless number of diseases that ruin their health. Nowadays, physicians are advising their patients to follow proper diet and regular exercise to regain health and fitness. Exercise or activities are of different types and one has to follow them according to their energy levels and physical stamina.

What Is Yoga?

There are different types of exercise regimens that include activities like aerobics, weight training, Pilates and so on. Yoga can be defined as one such exercise program which is quite different from others. It is a kind of science that has several branches and categories. Yoga is native to the land of India where it was discovered thousands of years ago. The word Yoga is derived from the language Sanskrit and it means "the union". The art of yoga implies the union of mind and body and also the union of soul with the mind. With the practice of yoga when these three entities; body, mind and soul are united it leads to several positive changes in an individual. Good health and fitness is one of the several changes that it brings. Yoga activates the purification process of our body and mind. It helps the body in automatically rejecting all the negativities that clog the progress and development of our body as well as mind.

The Practice Of Yoga

1. Yoga is a special program that comprises of different poses or Asanas. Attaining these poses is sometimes difficult. However, a practitioner of yoga has to attain various poses and maintain it for few seconds or few minutes to complete the activity of Yoga.

2. Along with poses, Yoga involves breath control, breathing exercises and meditation. These three aspects are sometimes practiced together and sometimes separately.

3. There are three levels or stages of Yoga. Practice of Yoga primarily helps in the physical development of a person. It reduces the influence of various diseases and prevents the occurrence of a wide range of ailments. It strengthens the body and improves its immunity power.

4. Practice of Yoga helps in controlling one's mind. It reduces the randomness of the mind and helps in making the mind more stable and more strong. It helps the mind in purifying itself by eliminating all the negative thoughts. Thus it leads to mental peace.

5. Practice of Yoga also helps in spiritual awakening. However, this stage is attained by dedicated practitioners only. By purifying the mind, Yoga helps the mind to fixate on its consciousness about the self or the soul. This gradually leads to a divine form of spiritual development. Such practitioners develop a strong aura around themselves and their faces grow brighter and more lustrous.

6. In order practice Yoga, one needs to have a teacher or a Guru. Yoga should be practiced as per the instructions given by a certified Yoga master. Self practice can lead to mistakes that can cause severe side effects. Hence, it is advised in general to avoid the practice of yoga in the absence of a teacher or an instructor.

7. There are several videos and movies published by various Yoga experts that show how various Yoga postures and poses should be done. You can follow such methods to begin with basic Yoga practice. However, advanced Yoga which includes practices like "Pranayama" should never be practiced in the absence of a master or Guru.

8. Practice of Yoga should be undertaken in the early morning or in the evening hours. You should practice Yoga only with an empty stomach. After a meal you should wait for 4 hours in order to practice Yoga. After practicing Yoga you should not consume any food for another 1 hour. However, there is no restriction for drinking water, juices or milk.

9. When you are practicing Yoga, you should keep your mind clam and peaceful. There is no point in practicing Yoga with a disturbed or preoccupied mind.

10. While practicing yoga, you should wear loose clothes. Do not wear clothes that restrict your body movement or that cause discomfort to your body or skin.

11. Yoga should be practiced in a peaceful and open environment. You can also practice it in a room that has good ventilation. Good oxygen supply enhances the effects of different Yoga steps.

12. Yoga practice should be undertaken in a peaceful environment. Loud noises and harsh music should be avoided when you are practicing yoga.

13. Do not practice Yoga when you are exhausted, tired or sick. You should be physically and mentally comfortable when you are doing Yoga.

14. While doing Yoga, if you feel too exhausted or stressed, then you should wait for sometime before resuming.

15. Certain Yoga poses are too difficult to practice. Obese people find it difficult to stretch their limbs beyond a limit. In such cases, one should not try hard to make the pose perfect. This can hurt your body. You should realize that it can take days or even months to perfect a pose or an 'Asana'.

16. Always use a mat made of cloth or straw in order to practice Yoga. Never practice yoga directly on the floor. This can hurt your tissues. Moreover, when you are practicing Yoga, lots of energy flows through your body. In order to retain the energy within your body you should make use of a substance that doesn't absorb energy. If you do it on

the floor, the energy will be transmitted down from your feet onto the floor.

17. Drink water before doing Yoga. Water is necessary for proper cell function. Water will allow the muscles to stretch comfortably.

Basic Yoga practices include poses or Asanas that can be practiced by anyone without any restriction. However, people suffering from spine injuries should avoid these since they might hurt their spine.

1. Hastapadasana :

Hastapadasana is a basic pose or Asana that involves stretching of arms and thighs. Hasta means hand and Pada means feet.

- In this Asana, you need to bring your hands near to your feet. You should stand straight and then bow down from your waist until your hands touch the toes of your feet.

- While bending you should keep your knees straight. There is no point in bending your knees and bringing your hand close to your feet. Slowly, stretch your hands and place your palms on either side of both the feet. Keep your breathing steady.

- This is a basic Asana that has several benefits. It reduces obesity and improves blood circulation to the head. It reduces hair fall. And it is also beneficial for our nervous system.

- Obese people may find it difficult to bring their hands near the feet. They should not exert any extra effort. They should stretch the hands as far as they can and let them remain that way for 1 or 2 minutes before leaving the pose.

2. Padma Asana:

Padma Asana is a basic pose in Yoga in which the body of a person resembles a lotus flower. Padma means lotus.

- In Padma Asana you should sit on the floor and fold both your legs and cross them over each other.

- Now slowly pull your right foot from between the folded left leg and place it against the left thigh. The sole of the foot should be facing upward. Repeat the same with the left foot too.

- Keep your hands near the knees and try to relax.

- These Asana strengthens the feet and thigh muscles. It has several benefits and it helps the body in many ways.

3. Matsya Asana:

Matsya Asana comes as a supine pose. The word Matsya means fish. In this Asana, the pose of the body resembles that of a fish.

- Lie down on your back. Cross both the legs just like you did for Padma Asana. Just cross the legs and there is no need to place the feet over the thighs.

- Lift both your arms and bend them backwards towards your head. Place your palms on the floor right next to your ears.
- With the support of your hands, lift the head and gently turn it backwards. Rotate your head until the chin points in the direction of the sky. Gently lower the head until it touches the floor.

- Once the head is placed on the floor, remove the hands and slowly bring them near your torso. Place the hands on your thighs.

- Remain in this pose for 1 minute.

- Slowly, release the pose. First move the arms backwards towards the head. Place the palms on the floor and by putting your weight on the palms slowly lift your head and rotate it back to its original position.

- Rest your head and then bring your hands back to its original position.

- Straighten the legs and relax for a minute.

- This Asana helps in reducing obesity. It helps in curing diabetes, malabsorption, sinusitis, asthma, bronchitis, colitis, sore throat and jaundice.

4. Hala Asana:

Asana is a difficult pose for the beginners. However, it can be done as best as you can. Since it is one of the most beneficial Asanas it is recommended by most of the Yoga Gurus. The word Hala means the 'plough'. Upon performing this Asana, the body assumes the shape of a traditional plough. For this reason it is named as Hala Asana.

- Lie down on your back, place the arms on your sides.

- Slowly lift both the legs together and bring them in 90 degree angle to the body.

- Support your hip with both your hands and slowly raise your hip

- Simultaneously, bend your legs right over your upper body and keep doing it until your feet touches the ground. At this time your entire hip will be in the air. Keep supporting your back with your hands.

- Remain in this position for a minute.

- Then slowly lift your legs and bring them to 90 degree angle. Slowly lower your hip until it touches the ground.

- Now lower your legs back to their original position.

- Keep both the hands on either side of the body and relax for a minute.

- This Asana helps in curing backache, sciatica, sexual debility, bronchitis, congestion, asthma, depression, headache, rheumatoid arthritis, sinusitis, premenstrual tension and so on.

5. Paschimothana Asana:

This Asana comprises of a forward bend. It is a simple Asana.

- Sit on the floor and spread both the legs straight.

- Keep the feet together. Now, slowly lift your arms straight up.

- Bring down your arms but keep them straight. Along with your arms bend your whole body.

- Keep bending until your hands touch your feet.

- Hold the feet or the toes with your fingers.

- Keep your knees straight while doing this.

- Obese people might find it a bit difficult to touch their feet. However, it is not recommended to overstretch your arms or body. Do as best as you can and leave it at that.

- After a minute slowly raise your arms up and raise your whole torso. Raise the arms up and slowly move them sideways to lower them.

- Releasing a pose is as important as doing a pose. So, it is imperative that you follow these instructions closely.

- This Asana helps in reducing the fat deposits near the waistline. It helps in trimming the arms and thighs. It also strengthens the muscles of your back and arms.

6. Bhujanga Asana:

Bhujanga Asana is a basic pose which is practiced by lying on your belly. The word Bhujanga means snake or serpent. In this Asana, the body acquires a serpent like position with its head raised up in the air.

- Lie down on your belly with your arms on either side of your body
  - .

- Slowly bring your hands up and place them on either side of your face.

- Place your palms on the floor and support your torso.

- Slowly lift your torso and head upwards from the waist.

- While raising your body take a deep breath.

- Raise your head up until your face points in the direction of the sky.

- Once you reach this position start exhaling slowly.

- Keep the legs straight and keep your feet pointed towards the sides.

- Remain in this position for a minute and then slowly begin to lower your torso.
- Slowly retain the original position and then retreat your hands down on either side.

- This Asana helps in improving blood circulation in the spine area. It is beneficial to the upper parts of your body including your stomach.

- It is a very good stretching exercise for the arms and torso.

- For women this Asana helps in curing menstrual problems. It is also beneficial for the ovaries and the uterus. The Asana also promotes easy child birth. However, do not practice this Asana during pregnancy.

7. Dhanur Asana:

Dhanur Asana is quite popular for reducing the fat stores around the abdomen. Dhanur in Sanskrit means "bow". In Dhanur Asana, the body assumes a shape that resembles a bow.

- To perform Dhanur Asana lie down on your belly and keep your arms on either side.

- Bend the legs at the knees and stretch your arms and try to reach your feet.

- Stretch the arms and hold the feet by their ankles. This will automatically raise the legs and the upper body above the floor level. The only part that touches the floor will be your abdomen.

- Raise your head and look upwards. Remain in this position for 1 or 2 minutes.

- Slowly release the feet and lower the legs and arms to their original position.

- This Asana helps in strengthening the muscles of the abdomen and spine.

- It also helps in improving your posture.

- Reduces obesity.

- It strengthens the reproductive and digestive systems.

- It helps in curing bronchitis, constipation, rheumatism, asthma and diabetes.

8. Shalabha Asana:

Shalabha Asana is a simple and basic Asana that has several benefits. The word Shalabha means butterfly. The pose resembles the shape of a butterfly.

- Lie down on your belly. Keep your arms close to your body and relax.

- Your chin should be touching the floor.

- Keep both the legs close and slowly raise them by keeping the knees straight.

- Raise the legs around 30 degrees from the floor and remain in this position for 1 minute.

- Slowly lower the legs and resume the original position.

- This Asana helps in curing back pain, varicose veins and sciatica pain.

- It also cures constipation and indigestion.

- It helps in reducing obesity.

- It also helps in curing diabetes.

9. Ardha Matsyendra Asana:

This Asana is a bit complex but it has several benefits.

- Sit down on the floor with both the legs stretched out.

- Cross your right leg over your left leg and bend at the knee.

- Bend the left leg inwards and keep it close to the body.

- Reach with your left hand and try to hold your right big toe.

- While reaching out your left hand you should stretch the arm across the outer side of your right knee.

- Twist your torso to the right side and turn your head backwards.

- Also fold your right hand across the back.

- Remain in this position for 1 minute.

- Slow release your toes and straighten your arms. Also straighten your torso and look straight.

- Straighten your left leg and then lift your right leg and place it straight on the floor.

- You can repeat the entire pose by alternating the sides.

- It helps in reducing abdominal fat.

- It strengthens your pancreas, spleen, kidneys and liver.

- It cures indigestion.

- It strengthens the ligaments and spinal nerves.

10. Trikona Asana:

This Asana helps in stretching the whole body. Trikona means triangle. While doing this Asana, your body will assume a triangle-like shape.

- Stand straight and extend your left leg to one side.

- Slowly lean down and try to touch your left foot with your left hand.

- Stretch your right arm and point your right hand towards the sky.

- Turn your head and look in the direction of your right hand.

- Stay in this position for 1 minute.

- Now lower your right arm and slowly straighten your body.

- Slide your left leg back to its original position.

- Now you can repeat the same pose by alternating the sides.

- It helps in toning and strengthening the spinal nerves.

- It helps in curing indigestion.

11.Pawanmuktasana:

This Asana is quite simple to practice. It helps in releasing the air trapped within your abdomen.

- Lie down on your back and keep your legs straight.

- Lift your legs slowly and raise it at 60 degree angle.

- Bend your legs at the knees and raise them to your torso.

- Hold your knees close to your upper abdomen and hug your legs with both your arms.

- Press the legs closer to your body and gently raise your head.

- Lower you head back to its original position.

- Stay in this position for 1 minute.

- Now slowly release your arms and straighten your legs.

- Lower your legs back to the floor.

- Relax your body.

- This Asana helps in curing indigestion and constipation.

- It promotes appetite and removes flatulence.

- It strengthens your liver, spleen, stomach, urinary bladder and intestines.

12. Learning Surya Namaskara (Sun Salutation)

Surya Namaskara is one of the most important parts of Yoga. It is a series of poses that can be combined into a Salutation-like action. Traditionally, it was performed to please the Sun God. It includes 12 poses and on each step the practitioner has to say certain Mantra or the name of the Sun God.

Steps To Perform Surya Namaskara

1. Stand straight facing eastwards. Join both your hands in a prayer position. Raise both your arms and stretch your body. Now bend downwards and touch your feet.

2. Next, bend your right leg and stretch your left leg backwards. Place your hands on the floor and lower your entire body.

3. Support your entire body on both your arms and right leg and look upwards.

4. Now lift your body and straighten your right leg and place it alongside your left leg. Keep your hands on the floor itself. Bend your whole body at the hip level and point your torso downwards.

5. Now lower your hip and straighten your body. Also lower your head. Slowly place the whole body on the floor and now gently lift up your head and torso supported by your arms.

6. Now reverse back all the positions. Lift your torso and legs and bend your body at the hip level. Once again your torso will be pointing downwards. And your head will also be pointing down. Now bend your right leg at the knee and shift it forward.

7. Look upwards and turn your torso in the upper direction. Keep the left leg stretched and straight.

Your hands should be still on the floor for proper support.

8. Now come to a standing position but keep your torso bend. Keep both your hands next to your feet. Keep the body bent at the waistline.

9. Slowly rise up and also raise your arms upwards. Bend your body a bit backwards as you stretch the entire body.

10. Now lower your arms, straighten your back and join your hands in the prayer position, close to your torso. Now you are back to your first position from where you started.

This is the entire cycle of a single Sun Salutation. You can repeat it 12 times to get a good effect. This entire exercise is quite beneficial for reducing weight, improving your flexibility and for promoting digestion. It also strengthens your musculoskeletal system, nervous system and spine. It would be beneficial if you practice it in the morning. You can also practice it in the evening. However, it is better to practice it before sunset.

Relevance Of Finding A Teacher

1. For practicing yoga you need a good teacher. Although you can follow the instructions shown in videos and tutorials, it would be more beneficial if there is a teacher who can guide you depending on your pace and Yogic skills.

2. If you have a teacher, he or she can teach you advanced Yoga practices. This will help you in gaining more benefits from this famous art.

3. Once you learn under the guidance of a teacher, you will be apt enough to provide training to others. Thus, you can start your own Yoga class in future.

www.ingramcontent.com/pod-product-compliance
Lightning Source LLC
Chambersburg PA
CBHW072013280526
45788CB00005B/2028